I'll Be All Right Tomorrow

By

DYMPNA BROGAN

I dedicate this book to my family and friends as well as those in the caring professions who by their care and patience have made today possible.

This CreateSpace edition published in February 2015

First published in paperback in June 1999 by

>The Verbal Arts Centre
>
>Bishop Street Within
>
>Derry/Londonderry
>
>Northern Ireland
>
>BT48 6PU

Copyright © Dympna Brogan. All rights reserved

Front Cover Painting and drawings by Dympna Brogan

CreateSpace design by Vincent Brogan
info@tyroneroots.com

Originally published in paperback with assistance from The Roald Dahl Foundation

Foreword

This book came about because of various articles written by me which describe how I coped after a very serious accident. It took me a year to write this small book and it would not have been written if it were not for the skill and perseverance of my tutor, Hugh McGovern.

I went each week to the Adult Basic Education Department of Omagh College of Further Education with two pages and then Hugh and I would talk about the part in my life outlined in my two pages. From there we turned to the script, expanding, eliminating, re-arranging, adding and correcting. So I returned home with my two pages and a string of changes and rewrote my script once more.

This process continued until a first finished copy was completed. Then we took it again and eliminated repeated material and touched up the work. It was now no longer a workpad with changes and corrections but a complete book. At this point I was offered help by The Verbal Arts Centre, Derry.

I wish to especially thank Tricia Kelly for her perseverance and her persistence is securing funding from the Roald Dahl Foundation for publishing and printing the paperback version of this book.

I will never be an author but I felt I had a story to tell about how I felt when I had no control over my life and not a dozen words in my head to express myself. The writing of this book has been a great release of my feelings and a therapy in itself.

Dympna Brogan

June 1999

Contents

The Open Road	7
Trapped Inside My Head	14
'I will be your speech therapist'	22
Lover's Retreat	28
Rosaleen and Theresa	36
Vincent	42
Birth and Death	52
E For Epilepsy	58
Facing it	64
Talking to John	73
Now	79
Postscript to 2015 edition	85

One

The Open Road

'Are you sure you want to go? asked John. 'Of course', I replied as I settled myself comfortably into my seat. John slipped into the driver's seat and we were off through that wet February night towards Lisburn. It was 1974 and I was a student of Occupational Therapy at Jordanstown Polytechnic where John was a lecturer in Speech and Drama.

'Look out! I called

'At what? answered John as we rounded the bend, over the white line.

'Look out! Look out! I screamed.

On the other side of that bend a white van with two men inside came flashing towards us. There was panic and slamming of brakes and the white van crashed into the Morris Minor in which I was the front seat passenger. The force of the impact smashed my head against the side panel of the car.

After that a great series of activities began: phone calls, sirens, ambulances with their crews arriving, people helping, firemen, policemen and a nurse, lights flashing and figures moving among the shadows on the wet roadside – but of all these events I remember almost nothing at all. I do remember looking out through the tangled mass of twisted metal, oblivious of my own predicament and concerned only for the safety of my companion.

'Where is John?' I frantically asked.

'He is here,' the calm voice of an ambulance man replied.

'Is he all right?' Where are we going? I asked, as they lifted my body, slid a white stretcher beneath me and placed blankets over me.

'Is he all right? Is he all right? Is anything broken?' No one answered my shouts. I looked out at the night sky as they placed me inside the ambulance. John was brought in on the other side. He did not call out; his mouth was slightly open and his teeth were clenched. His eyes were closed very tightly and his hands were inside the white blankets.

'Are you all right?' I called out to him.

'I'm...I'm...OK'. His voice was barely audible. 'Open your mouth', ordered a nurse who seemed to appear out of nowhere. I obeyed and soon light began to fade and I slid into nothingness.

I awakened fitfully to blurred sounds and awareness of growing light. A small brown bird landed on the tree outside my window. I was snug and warm inside my bed in the Royal Victoria Hospital. I recognised the place because I had been a student nurse there the previous year. Now I was back in the same hospital.

The small bird was chirping on the tree outside. He was very active, flitting from branch to branch, now upright, now hanging upside down, inspecting, searching, feeding, always moving. I felt strangely immobile. What has happened? My blonde hair from the side of my head to my temple was shaved off and there were three tubes inserted into my wrists. I felt very hungry, I needed to talk to a nurse, I wanted to call out – why were there no words coming from my mouth?

'God,' - what was that word?

Eventually a nurse came.

'God,' I spluttered.

'Now, now, you will be all right. Do you want to go to the toilet?.

'God, God.' I tried to get out of bed, forgetting about the tubes.

'Wait! Wait! Hold on; please get back into bed,' I was told as panic struck the face of the student nurse. 'I will get you a bed pan,' she said.

'God.' Am I a geriatric now, twenty years old, no words to speak except 'God'? I am pinned to the bed, half my hair shaved off! What will I do when the dreaded visiting time arrives? 'God,' I will say, 'bloody God.' I wet myself before the nurse came with the bed pan.

The dreaded time came. The visitors from home arrived, my mother, my brother Pat and his fiancée, Lizzy. Mother was crying as she came up to my bed and the engaged couple held hands. 'Great to see you awake,' said Pat, smiling. 'you were asleep for eleven days.'

'God,' I answered.

'Can you not eat, Dympy?' asked Mum, as she got another tissue from her brown coat pocket.

'God.'

'Are you going to say nothing but God?' puzzled Pat.

'God' – as the saliva trickled down the side of my chin.

'Dear God,' Mother sobbed.

Another tissue was called for. They stood there uneasy.

Conversation was rapidly becoming burdensome, talk a stumbling block. There was a great silence.

'It's great to see you're awake,' said Pat, clenching Lizzy's hand. Pat was in a state of growing shock, aware that matters were much worse than he had suspected. He needed a respite. 'Must go – long way home.' Mother was still crying as she left the bedside.

Everyone in Omagh will know it now. They will know I cannot bloody speak. What has happened to my right side? I cannot raise my right arm, never mind opening and closing my right hand. The hospital routine did not allow any room for crying. My world had fallen around me in one minute. I buried my head in the blankets. I did not want to know myself. It was dark outside and the rain was falling.

I learnt later that my elder sister Kate who was at this time in England at a Teacher Training College in Leeds had come to visit me in Intensive Care. As soon as she heard about the accident she was granted five days leave of absence to come home. When she arrived at the hospital no one warned her of my condition before she entered the ward. She walked up to my bed, and then stopped in her tracks, aghast to see me wired up, corpse-like, motionless, wax-like pale, completely changed, barely recognisable. Kate stood there as if in a trance, trying to catch her breath. The ward sister came across to her at the bedside. 'Are you Miss Garrity?' she enquired.

'Yes,' said Kate, looking up slowly from the other side.

The sister shuffled uneasily. 'Because of the interior damage to the brain she will not be able to function normally again.'

'What?'

'The damage is very extensive.'

Not function normally...very extensive... Kate pondered the doom-laden words. 'I am sorry.'

Kate was still. She made no other reply. The ward sister stood a while in silence then she made some excuse and left. Kate sat on, stunned and wordless, bludgeoned by the avalanche of disastrous information. She did not attempt to speak to the figure she saw before her in the bed but was trying to come to terms with my present state and her own shock. After three hours she gathered her things together and left to spend a restless night with friends in Belfast. The next day, with courage restored, she came to see me again, hoping and hoping that some contact could be made. She felt that I knew that she was present, encouraged me to get well again, assuring me that I would get well, reminding me of past events and people, trying all the time to penetrate the far recesses of my memory store and kindle some spark of recognition. She asked me questions about myself even though she knew that I could not answer; she told me news which she hoped might interest me and maybe even stir me back to consciousness. With talk and spaces of silence she spent hours with me until time was up.

As she took my hand to say goodbye when time to go had come, she bent down and whispered, 'you will get better.'

Then she placed her hand in mine to take her leave and to her great surprise she felt me squeeze her hand. This was a great reward – great news – and she was happy: it was more than she had expected. Fortune was on the turn and there was hope.

There was nothing else that she could do for me in hospital, where all my needs were catered for. Two of her five days leave were gone so Kate thought it better to head for Killyclogher and home. She had some good news to take with her and it was important to tell Mum that there was a glimmer of hope.

Kate took the bus and started on her way to Omagh. Once at home she found it difficult to get around as there was no car. Mother was in a not-too-positive mood, which was not unusual. She drew tensely on her cigarettes. 'What's going to happen to wee Dympy?'

'Wee Dympy will be all right,' answered Kate abruptly.

'What's going to happen to me?' If she cannot look after herself I won't be able to do it. I couldn't!' Mummy cried.

'She will be all right,' said Kate, pressing a used tissue into Mum's hand. 'You wait and see.'

Kate stayed with Mum for the few days that were left to her and then returned to Leeds and her studies.

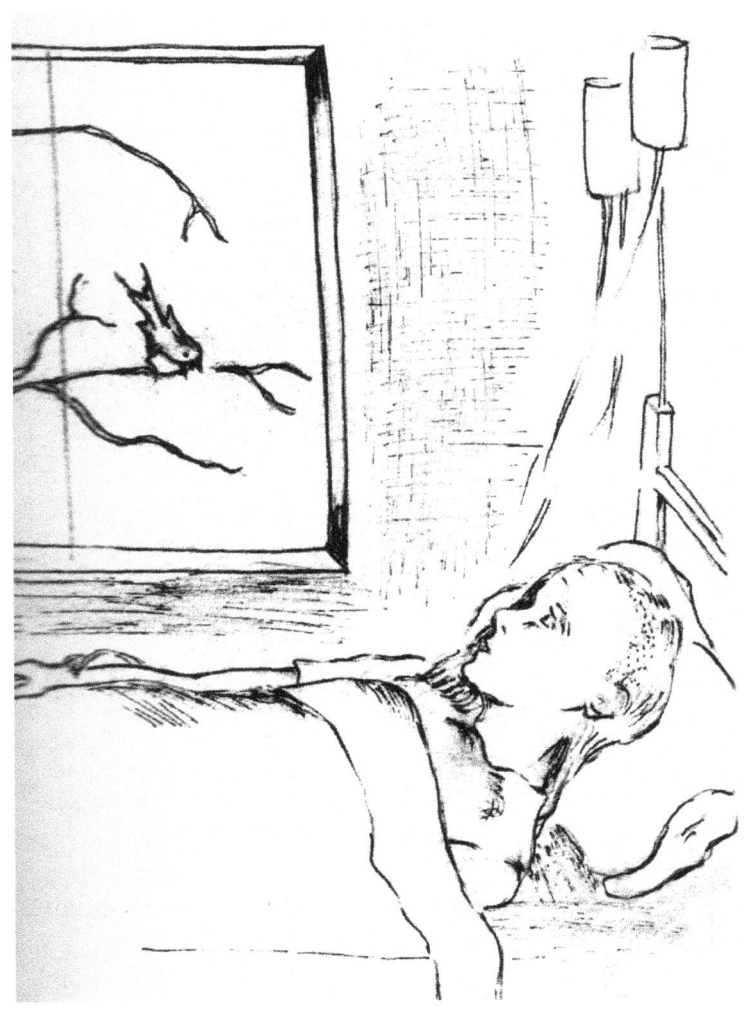

I felt strangely immobile

Two

Trapped Inside My Head

'Put your feet out of bed please, Dympna,' the nurse said. I was curled up like a snail. The student nurse repeated her request. I did not want to hear. I was trapped inside my head and the only word I could say was 'God'.

'Please Miss Garrity' said the student nurse, as she physically put my right leg over the bed. I tried to get up. What on earth was I wearing? My lovely black cotton coat which I had embroidered so beautifully, my black trousers, where are they now? I fell back into bed again. 'We will try again' the nurse said resignedly. I felt my arm. What sort of body had I woken up to? I was thin, which was not so before. I used to quite plump. I smiled and tried again and this time we got up. The nurse held my right hand the way I was taught the year before to hold a patient who for one reason or another could not help himself. I tried to recall the name of the hold as I dragged my right leg after me across the room but could not.

'Hello, Dympna,' whispered Brian; I was upset because you were not at the show on Friday night.'

'God.'

'We can work with God. Actually I was talking to him before I came out to see you,' he said lightly.

I laughed and his face lit up to see a smile on my face.

Brian was an actor and at the time had a part in the chorus of *Jesus Christ Superstar* at the Lyric Theatre.

'I must get his autograph for you,' he joked.

Brian came up every day of my stay at the hospital. Later I learned that he felt responsible for my injuries because he did not know the exact date of the accident. He thought that the accident had happened when I was coming to see the show but it had taken place on the night before. His visits helped me. He talked to me and humoured me and I loved him for that.

Now the visitors came in thick and fast to see me. Some came and talked to other visitors who came to see me. There I lay dribbling away saying 'God, God'. An old boyfriend, Vincent, arrived. He had a book with him, perhaps it was for me. He looked at me and a shocked expression spread across his face. He stood about for some time and said little. When he left, the book was sitting on the table. I got it into my hand, fumbled it open and looked inside: it was a book of poetry.

He knew I liked poetry and it was good of him to bring what pleased me and I was grateful. But, my God, when I looked inside, the whole thing was jumbled up – the shapes of words were lost, the pattern of print was gone, the page was a maze of strokes and slashes, a meaningless jumble. I had made another discovery about myself. I cannot speak and now I cannot read. I thought, this is terrible! I got out of bed and desperately hunted around the room searching for a pen. At last I found one and tried it out. I wrote the word 'the'. Now my name? What is my name? I cannot remember my own name! I went over to my bed and closed the curtains, sat down on a chair and began to cry silently.

I cannot read or write, I cannot talk. I had tried so desperately before to attain my level of literacy. While classmates had skated effortlessly along through the school programme, I had survived, only by striving and hard work and now it had all vanished I did not want to start again.

What was there to look for; what was there to live for? I did not want to live. I wanted to die. My life before was talking, moving, expecting, exploring, expanding relations, doing things, conversation and discussion. Now there was nothing. I wanted to die but how could I commit suicide in the hospital? The drugs were under lock and key. How about drowning?

I gathered up my toiletry things, went to the bathroom and locked myself inside. I turned on the shower and held my face at the correct angle to die. I remembered from biology lessons how the oesophagus muscle closes to prevent food and liquid entering the lung chamber. The water flowed across my face, poured into my mouth and nose but the muscle closed the way into my lungs. Why did my body not agree with my head? I lay down on the floor and cried myself tired. Nothing was happening but the constant falling of water all over me and the small sounds of comings and goings. Outside there were occasional sounds of footsteps, of a door closing or, sometimes, the muffled sounds of the city beyond the hospital walls but they all seemed to belong to a world very far away from me.

'Are you coming for your supper?' shouted a staff nurse.

The voice was firm and authoritative. I knew what was expected. A hospital is a place of business, order and obedience.

'God,' I sobbed. I got myself up from the floor, gathered up my things and went for my supper. The hospital routine rolled on regardless.

That night an elderly gentleman visited me. He looked a kind, considerate, caring sort of a man. 'My name is Mr Walton and I was your surgeon, Dympna.' He spoke to me in a calm, quiet way. 'It's great to see you awake. 'I sat up in bed.

'Can I sit down and tell you what happened?'

'Oh, please, yes!' I wanted to say but only 'God' came out.

'Because of the impact, the carotid artery was blocked in your neck. That meant lack of oxygen to the temporal lobe part of your brain – you have brain damage, Dympna.'

'God!' I gasped.

'You have three holes in the side of your head because we needed to remove the excess fluid from the interior of the brain.'

'Oh God!'

We sat still for some time.

'You won't be able to talk now. Do you know how long you were unconscious?'

'God.'

'Eleven days.'

I nodded.

'Also, your right side is paralysed because of the injury to your brain.'

Another silence followed.

'Can you swim?'

I shook my head.

'Can you float?'

I nodded my head.

'It is important that you first float at this particular time, Dympna.'

'God'.

He sat on as darkness gathered outside the window and the night staff began to drift into the wards checking patients and bed charts.

He stood up. 'It's quite late now. I will see you again. Good night.'

I nodded my head and as the elderly gentleman was going through the door, I noticed that he was limping. For the first time I understood what had happened to me and I felt grateful to him.

I cannot remember how long it was before therapy began.

The Occupational Therapy Unit was in a small room somewhere in the new part of the hospital. They wanted me to ride a stationary cycle. I remember thinking how humiliating it was to be on the receiving end rather than the giving end of occupational therapy. I wanted to be my old self;

Dympna Garrity
Student of Occupational Therapy
Jordanstown Polytechnic

My thoughts drifted back to that time. How I wished to be back there. In 1973 a new exciting course was being introduced in Jordanstown. This was in Occupational Therapy under the guidance of Miss Joy Rook. We were the first to embark upon that course, myself and eighteen other girls. I at twenty years of age was the 'Mammy' of the group. It was fantastic! What had happened before in my life was tame and common compared to this. This place was huge, spectacular, exciting, with freshness and newness all about. It had buzz. I was liberated, an adult, treated as an adult, in an adult world, responsible to myself and free. There was in the course a sense of present and future achievement and I loved every part of all I felt and saw. Miss Rook was a woman of courage and frankness who sometimes took us by surprise. 'What is wrong with me?' asked Miss Rook one day in first term. I was very near to where she was sitting. We were very surprised at such a strange question. There was no response. After a short silence she repeated the question. Again there was no reply. She shifted in her seat and held up her hand in open view. 'Now can you see?' Part of a finger of her right hand was missing. 'No one is perfect,' she said. 'Everyone has something wrong with them, physically or mentally.' She was a lecturer who was not afraid of opening up her own wounds. Remembering those times I thought about how the tables had turned now. The three lecturers from the polytechnic came to see me, Miss Gardiner, Miss Sage and Miss Rook. The frankness of Miss Rook impressed me strongly at the time and when she came to visit me accompanied by Miss Gardiner and Miss Sage I recalled her courage. Here was I, student of the first group to study occupational therapy and now I felt only acute embarrassment to find myself in a hospital bed before my tutors and without the power to speak to them. By this time I was able to move without aid from anyone. Some good person had brought in my own clothes and it felt good to put them on and regain something of my old self. I wondered how the opposite sex would view me now, with my dripping mouth, my shorn head, not able to talk and with no power in my right hand. I felt as if my right side was gone from me because the feeling was not there. I wondered if I could still enjoy kissing or ever be passionately aroused again. This was not the place to be if I wanted to try out these experiments. The three basic human needs are for food, shelter and sex. I was a human female and my basic needs were the same. Being twenty years of age at the time I wanted everything to happen now, so I tried to masturbate in the middle of that same night. I hoped that no one saw me. The experiment was a success. At least the basic instincts were still intact.

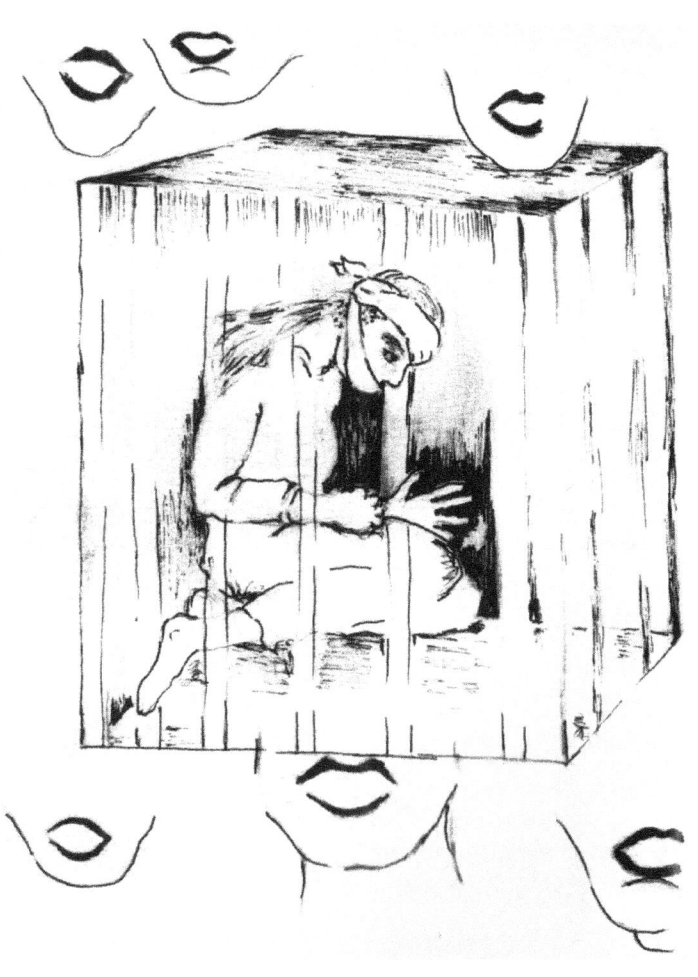

I was trapped inside my head

Three

'I will be your speech therapist'

'My name is Miss Key and I will be your speech therapist, Dympna.'
Before me was an elderly, plump lady who sat down behind her table when I had been wheeled up to her.
'Oh yes, oh yes, please help me, Miss Key,' I rushed to say but no words came. Miss key just talked calmly to me and I listened. Soon her words began to drift into the distance and I found my thoughts fixed on John. I had heard that he was a patient in Musgrave Park Hospital. I wanted to write to him a letter, wanted to know he was well, wanted to tell him that I was responsible for the accident and to let him know that I was thinking of him constantly. I would end, 'To John, with much love, Dympna.'

Miss Key was still speaking to me, her words drifting in and out of my consciousness. I suppose she knows about brain damage, about loss, confusion. One minute she has my whole attention, next minute my mind has gone off at a tangent or I am far away in my own world.

I did manage to get that letter written with the help of a nurse. It was not very readable but I thought that John would manage to decipher it and I hoped that he would be pleased. He eventually got the letter and years later he gave it back to me. So Miss Key proceeded with speech therapy, mostly speaking to me as I sat before her, greedily attentive or totally inattentive.

While Miss Key was trying to restore my speech for me a former boyfriend came to see me and talk to my eyes. He was Jack Mullan, a nurse from Purdysburn Hospital. Jack was a sturdy fellow with fair hair, blue eyes and a round face with a double chin. Jack spent his time with me trying to teach me how to relax: start at your toes, move your body, limb by limb, to the top of your head. It worked. After half an hour of this treatment my body – or should I say half of my body – was relaxed. I was grateful for his help and that he had come to see me and talk to me.

Meanwhile Miss Key was working hard with me. She was a kind, comforting, gentle lady who made me feel at ease. But I needed to talk, longed to talk, wanted desperately to talk. I was not going to let this terrible thing rob me of my speaking voice. My world of speech was lost to me in reality but sometimes in my daydreams a fantasy of this world came back to me and in these dreams the words flowed from me with great power and ease and marvellous fluency. I relished its joys but awoke to the real world where things happened slowly, painfully, one word at a time. Sometimes a word was with me for the whole day and then was gone. Sometimes a word was with me for a little while and then was gone. Sometimes an unusual word like 'epiglottis' or 'clavicle' came and stayed with me. Words kept coming and leaving, single words not accompanied by their associated words but there was no assurance that they would come to me when I called them to mind.

All this time I was extremely ashamed to be where I was, in hospital, unable to look after myself and then it happened. I was going home. I was being expelled! I had been about one month there in all. The curing was over, at least all that they were willing to do or could do. So that was that. Help was at an end and Miss Key and occupational therapy were of the past.

The expulsion took place on a Sunday and I went down in my brother Pat's car to the town of Omagh and from there to Mother's bungalow in the heart of the countryside. There I would be assured of having plenty to eat but it would also be sure that nothing much was likely to happen. To get around would be a problem. If Pat was not at work or if he was not courting he would be able to drive me but his time was limited. Kate returned at Easter and by then I was at home in limbo trying feverishly to get a start on my rehabilitation. Up to now there was nothing and my frustration was intense, and the turmoil in my life begun to infect the whole household.

Kate could and would help and she began by writing a set of alphabet flash cards. I could not distinguish the letters so I drew the pictures from the card before me. Kate took the cards and held them one by one before me and called out the letters. 'A...B...C...D.'

'AA...BB...CC...DD.'

Then she tried me on my own.

'A...B....'

After that there is nothing. My frustration is exploding. This is terrible, this is Primary One stuff; it is pre-school – it is playschool for God's sake!

'Fuck... fuck...fuck.. .'

Panic broke out. Mother rushed in from the kitchen. 'Don't do any more, Kate, can't you see what you've done?' Mother demanded angrily. Kate looked at her. 'But she wants me to!'

She held up a flash card:
'B,' she said.
I drew a bed.
'God,' I said.
'B.'
We proceeded on in our faltering way.
'You are doing very well' said Kate. 'Would you like to relax for a bit now?'

I picked up the flash cards and handed them to her pressing her to start again. I was ready; my hand was poised to do the drawing. I needed – I needed desperately to talk.

'C.'
I drew a cup.
'Great Dympna. 'D.'
I waited but nothing came to me.
'Fuck...fuck....'

This outburst shattered any sliver of peace that still existed in the house. 'Leave it! Leave it! Look what you've done again! Mum scolded. Kate looked about her, not knowing what to do, to heed Mum's demands or my demands – and they were poles apart. Her problem would solve itself soon when she would return to Leeds and her own affairs.

On Sunday afternoons it was often a custom with us to visit relations. On one such Sunday afternoon soon after I returned to Omagh we went visiting Aunt Dympna. Aunt Dympna was special to me because I had been named after her. She had been the first to visit my mother after I was born so to mark this, I was given her name. When anyone visited Aunt Dympna a warm welcome was assured. She was a thin, energetic woman who busied herself tidying, cleaning and improving her comfortable home and doing all the baking for her family. She said, 'l heard that you said "God" all the time. Isn't just great that you keep praying away!' At that particular time God was the least of my concerns but I had no desire to disillusion good Aunt Dympna.

After the pleasantries were exchanged the focus of conversation would start circulating around me and I did not want to take part so I decided to stay out of the kitchen. It was May time, two months after leaving hospital but still I was prevented from going anywhere alone. I always needed someone to go with me; I was under house arrest and it was choking me. Another Sunday we were visiting another relation,

Aunt Mary. Inside, again, the talk revolved around me. I heard all; I understood all but could not participate. It irritated me and I left.

Outside Aunt Mary's door stood her bicycle. It was an old black lady's bike. I looked at it a while and wondered if I could manage. The place round about was level and concreted. The others were inside; there was no danger of interference, no one to annoy me or prevent me: the way was clear. I gripped the handle bar with my good left hand and propped the bicycle against myself. Then with my left hand on the handle bar, got astride the bicycle and launched myself. I wobbled my way across the yard and arrived safely. Rosaleen my fourteen year-old sister, rushed into the house and shouted 'Dympna is riding a bike!' They all pressed out the back door to watch a twenty-year-old ride a bike. My first real spin was down the Fintona road. It was great! Transport was available to me now, on a bike. So journeys on my own began again, half a mile down to Killyclogher to buy a bottle of the cheapest sherry in McGinn's bar and take it home to drink with my Mummy.

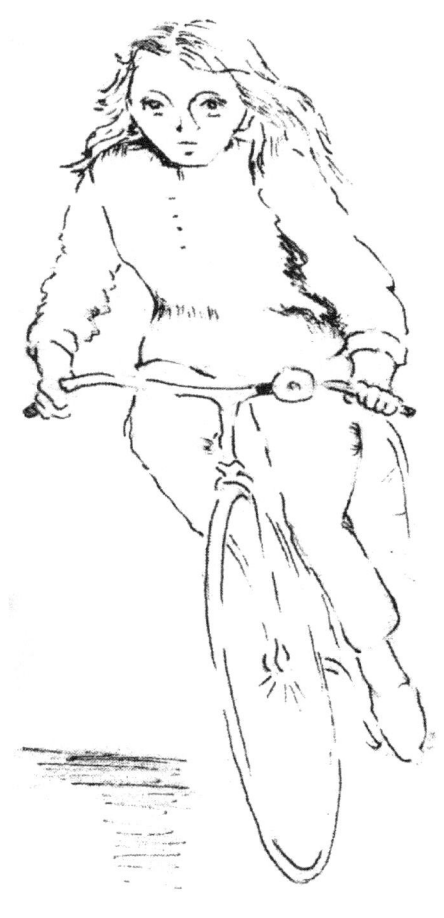

Four

Lovers' Retreat

There was no telephone, I couldn't write and so there were no methods of communication open to me. John was back at home in Lisburn and had kept in communication by letter. How embarrassing it was for me to have John's letters read to me by my mother. He wanted to see me, to come down to Omagh to visit me. So a date was set and he was taken down by his elderly parents, like a child, a back seat passenger in the family car – a far cry from what he was before, a lecturer in Speech and Drama at the polytechnic, an active man in the active role of drama teacher. His parents did not come into the house, making instead the excuse of having an appointment somewhere else. At the time I thought it was discourteous of them not to come into Mummy's house. I suspect now that they were familiar with the details of the accident and perhaps they thought John was responsible for the whole wretched mess, that they blamed him, and that it was now too uncomfortable for them to look at the results.

Nearby there was a pleasant wooded area by the river called Lovers' Retreat. It was much used by people out walking and I suggested that we should go there.

'I want to go too.' shouted Rosaleen.

'No you are not going,' Mummy said softly.

This was one of the most considerate remarks mother had made. She in some way understood our situation. I kissed her and we set off.

It was a grey May afternoon. John was now an invalid, stiff and thin, and walking like an old man, with the aid of a stick.

He did not know what to do with his free hand, whether to put it in mine or use it to support himself. It was strange to watch his face: he was happy to see me but distressed to see my state.

There was a tree in Lovers' Retreat, a weeping willow tree that I had known for years, one which I thought particularly beautiful. It was shaped like a horse and had one branch rising from the head like a fountain. With a majesty all of its own, it had become part of myself and I had drawn it with love. When we came to the place where it had stood we found it was no more. Someone from the Council had cut it down and concreted over the place where it had gown. The sight of this depressed me more than I can say. It had seemed a symbol of the present, of youth, beauty, energy, hope a little while ago – now we were two invalids pondering the past afraid of the future.

Now I wanted to comfort John to help him, to look after him and protect him by not telling how the accident had left me. I did not realise, even at that time, how grievously I was affected.

I remember thinking 'I'll be all right tomorrow,' and I believed that it would be so, that tomorrow would come one day, and my recovery, my restoration, my rehabilitation would arrive as quickly as my fall from grace. It was not going to be all right tomorrow but to believe so was of vital importance: it was a spur to make me do something, to strive today, every day. If I did nothing, nothing would happen. We spent a couple of hours of troubled companionship together and returned to

Mum's house, and from there John was taken back to Lisburn and I remained as before.

Meanwhile, some help was arranged locally. At four o'clock on a Tuesday afternoon an ambulance arrived and brought me to the swimming pool in Campsie. There were other patients picked up in and around Omagh and now I was one of the patients. How I detested that word. The water was lovely and warm and I had my own tutor. It was a relief to get out of the house, not to be forever wrapped in cotton wool in my mother's place, to be active at something. When I got in into the pool with Catherine, my tutor, I started to float. She was delighted that I could do this simple exercise: it was a start. She set out to teach me how to swim but as soon as she began I panicked. I did not know the right of me from the left of me. My right side was a foreign land to me; I was a paper doll sliced in two from top to bottom but I wanted to learn. I needed to learn, learn anything and I was desperately reaching out to someone who could help me on my way.

My brother Pat was trying to teach me to count from one to ten. 'One,' I managed, as I looked at Pat, who was having his dinner.

Pat was a joiner, a good joiner but no academic. Book learning had no draw for him. School had been a house of detention, a place from which one escaped to the real world of work. This was bewildering turn of fate that Pat should have become my tutor.

'After one what comes? 'Asked Pat.
'One after one?'
'One after one... what comes?'

He looked at me with kindness and questioning in his eyes.

'One, two, three – is that what you want to hear Dympna?' he asked.

Beaming, I set off again:

'One..one..one..one..fuck...fuck.'

Pat moved closer to me in the kitchen.

'Try it again, Dympna: one..two..three.'

'One..one..two..God.'

'Then three, Dympna.'

'One.. one.. one... fuck.. fuck... fuck.'

My face was in a snarl like an angry dog. My whole body was tense like a violin string, my eyes wild with rage. I did an O-level in maths three years ago and now I can't remember what comes after one.

'Now, now, now – what's the matter?' Mother interrupted, returning to the kitchen.

'One, one, two, two..' I blurted.

'Brilliant, Dympna!'

'After two?' asked Pat, starting his cold dinner once again.

'Can you not leave the counting aside a while?' asked mum.

Pat wanted to get on with his dinner and did not want to be interrupted any more.

'Two,' I repeated.

'A cup of tea, son?' said Mummy, as she came across to the table.

'Any niceties today, Mum?' Pat asked, looking up at her.

'Not today, Pat,' answered Mum sadly.

Outside the window it was high summer and the world was a sea of green and growing. I had no part in it.

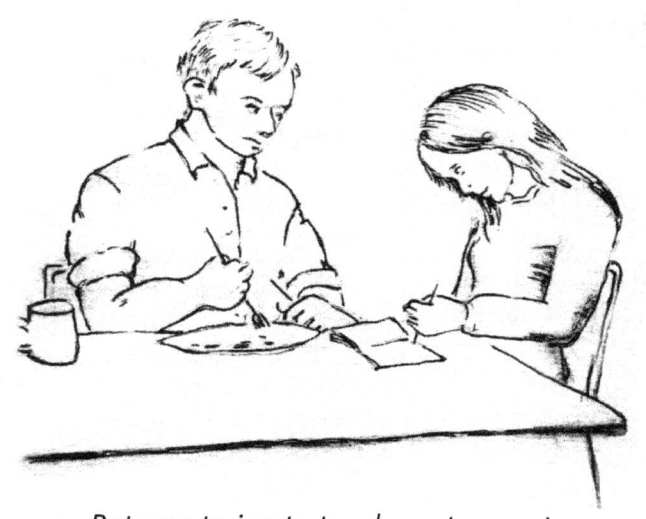

Pat was trying to teach me to count

Strangely, all this green and growing began to affect me positively. It became for me the spur for fresh effort, fresh thinking. Everywhere things were stretching out, trees, bushes, weeds and grass narrowing the green tunnels of country roads, closing paths. Everything was young and green getting out of its shell, breaking boundaries. Yes, I will break boundaries. I must break. I will get back to Belfast. Mother? God, she was good to me and cared for me, looked after my basic needs but accepted that the present was unchangeable; to witness my painful efforts at recovery was for her a torture, which then became an additional burden for me.

Yes, Belfast was my destination. The Troubles? I did not even think of them. Change needed to come. I needed my freedom as the bird coming out of its shell. In

Belfast there were speech therapists, physiotherapists, occupational therapists. If I got my speech back, reading and writing would soon follow. The people who could help me were in Belfast. Here there was nothing. I had friends in Belfast too and they would help. Quickly, the idea grew in my head until it became a fixation. Belfast became heaven to me, the be-all and end-all of all my thoughts. But how could I persuade Mummy to set me free? That would be a hard task; but in the end she would figure in the equation, for I was going no matter what.

I had been only five months at the polytechnic in Belfast, the honeymoon period, a wonderful place, marvellous place. We were all young and free and outgoing and there were fellas galore for the picking. For Mummy, my going there had been a leap into the dark and, worse, a leap into the Troubles. The Troubles were then at their peak and every day, morning, noon and night, televisions and radios were switched on so that we could find out what had happened in Belfast that day. Mother felt that to let me go there was to abandon me to strangers in a place of death, destruction and mayhem. She was not convinced when I told her that I had my friends there and professionals who would see me through. She could only see her daughter going into the unknown, quite helpless. Still the pinnacle of my desire was to be back in Belfast and in the end Mummy did not have any alternative but to let me go.

I set off for Belfast in Vincent's car with a happy heart. At last I was free of the restrictions of home and with two or three words for every sentence and getting better all the time. Soon, I thought, my speech would be back, reading and writing would follow and I would be back the way I was before, a student again at the polytechnic and the honeymoon resumed.

'I'll be all right tomorrow.'

My friends, who were as sound as my expectations suggested, immediately found a place for me among them and I began again to relish the old life. For many at that time Belfast might not have seemed a great place to live in but I felt great to be staying with my friends from Omagh in the 'Holy Land' off the Ormeau Road.

The schedule of therapies were about to begin and I would embrace them with great gusto. A month later and I was given a job as a helper in the occupational therapy department of the Royal Victoria Hospital. The job had been created for me by some kind person for my own therapy but this did not occur to me at the time. I still had ambitions to make a career in a caring role and now I had the opportunity to help elderly patients in my new work-cum-therapy job.

The job gave me stability and I felt that I was in control of my life again. If I did not want to go down home at the weekends I just did not take the bus. The routine of works, the demands of good timekeeping, which was never one of my brightest virtues, steadied me, although this was more a case of self-discipline as, if I was late, no one really complained. When the work made more demands on me than I could manage, I pretended that everything was normal and my work colleagues played the game along with me, helping me out, cheerfully and unobtrusively. They had the insight to realise that I was not able to cope with the accident and the baggage which had come along in its wake.

John kept in touch with me and visited me to see how I was getting along. He himself was now able to drive a car and was back in his old job in the polytechnic. I was determined that I would be back there too, come October. My perception was still that he needed me, needed to be protected by me, and could not do without my help. I was not in need of help. I could cope. Everyone else was a victim – except me.

I needed to be needed, very badly.

October came and fall of leaf. I still had a great difficulty with my speech. Nouns and verbs came most easily but the prepositions and joining words were more difficult. Sentences consisted of key words and when I managed to come up with all the words, they came in the wrong order.

'House I am going into.'

All the time I was haunted by the thought of what I was to do about my reading and writing problems. All through the summer months I had imagined that I would be back in the polytechnic by autumn, quietly picking up where I had left off. My language problems remained yet still I kept thinking to myself, 'I'll be all right tomorrow.' But October passed, the leaves fell and I was not back at the polytechnic.

Five

Rosaleen and Theresa

For four and a half years I worked in the Royal and at the end of that time I began to feel discontented. I had reached a plateau in my learning and felt that I was going nowhere. My ambition to succeed was however alive and well, and I was determined to do something about it. I had heard of a tutor called Miss Hill who had Adult Literacy classes in her own house. Her credentials were impeccable. She had been teaching English in a special care school in Belfast where her pupils received outstanding results in the O-level English examinations. 'Well, 'I thought, 'if you can do that for them, you can do it for me too.' So I left my job, signed up with Miss Hill and began to study hard, ferociously hard.

I rapidly became a workaholic. It had been my decision to leave my job, not one which had been forced on me from above, so I was not eligible for help from social security. So what? I had enough money, too much money. Settlement of the insurance claim had come through and I had been awarded £40,000. I had been unwilling to pursue a compensation claim, seeing it, I suppose, as an admission that I had suffered a permanent injury. Others had taken the process in hand on my behalf. I remember my solicitor handing me a cheque for £40,000 in 1977 and thinking, "That's an awful lot of money.' I took it, walked down the street and lodged it in the Ulster Bank. Then I set out down the town to spend it.

I bought a long pink nightdress at £6.00 and a good bargain it was too, as I have it still, nearly twenty years later, tucked away in my bottom drawer. I don't know what a learned psychologist might make of my first purchase but some of my friends found it funny and jokingly said it was a terrible extravagance. Another friend interpreted it as meaning that I was either a night owl or thrifty country lass making a start on her bottom drawer.

Monday, Wednesday and Thursday mornings now saw me beavering away under the guidance of Miss Hill. She knew how to set me homework and lots of it. Tuesdays and Fridays I worked as a Voluntary Helper with the NSPCC – from working with the elderly I had progressed to working with the 'wee ones'. My days were full of activity and in the evenings I was hammering away at Miss Hill's homework. I began to realise that any skills which I had before the accident had evaporated. I wanted to advance my skills and get back on to a ladder of learning that would give me a skill, any skill. Miss Hill and her homework were very important. When exam time came I was not ready and was not entered as a candidate.

In 1979 on a Friday evening, the eve of St Swithin's Day, I was getting ready to go home to Omagh for the weekend when I changed my mind at the last moment. I went off with some friends instead and got up quite late the next day. In the afternoon the telephone rang and I recognised the voice of Theresa, an old school friend, on the other end.

'Do you know what happened last night?' she asked.

'No,' I replied, puzzled. There was a long silence.

'Dympna, your sister Rosaleen drowned last night in the river at the Lover's Retreat.'

'No! No! No!'

'I will come up and collect you. I should be there in about two and a half hours. 'Thank you, Theresa,' I managed to answer. I put down the phone, sat down and felt the waves of shock pass over me. There was no one in the house; everyone had gone home or away for the weekend. Why had I not gone home? I had a friend around the corner and I needed to speak to someone so I went round to Paul's house. When I got there the place was empty too, so there was nothing for it but to go back to the house. When I entered our kitchen again in that friendly old house in Ireton Street I kicked the white back door as violently as I could.

When I arrived home, Mummy was there and began to tell me how things had happened; she spoke in a stunned, hypnotic manner. 'When you did not arrive home, Dympy, Rosaleen went off by herself. A wee boy found her.. drowned.. in The Lover's Retreat.. near the water's edge...She had picked flowers... near the water's edge.' When she had finished she began sobbing deeply.

Rosaleen did not have any scars on her when I saw her lying in her coffin. She had a blue shroud on and her hands were clasped as if in prayer. Her face was white, her eyes closed. Her mouth was smiling. When I felt her hands they were cold. She was dead.

There was one night of a wake. Rosaleen was the youngest and the pet of the family. Since childhood she had suffered from epileptic fits and as she grew older the attacks had become more severe and more frequent. This was a continual worry for her and for all the family. The physical dangers of an attack, especially if she had one when no one else was around, preyed on all our minds. The condition was robbing her of her independence, preventing her from having a life of her own. Now Rosaleen, the youngest, was dead and buried at nineteen years old.

    I was fifteen years old when my father died and after his death we moved house. Now after the death of Rosaleen we moved again. We had moved several times around the Omagh area so now we began to feel like nomads. How was all this going to affect Mummy, I wondered – how was it all going to affect me? Where was my place in the new equation? My brother Pat was married and had small children so he had his own responsibilities. Kate my other sister was teaching in England. I knew what Mummy wanted. She didn't breathe a word about it but I could read the message in her eyes. Her eyes said, 'Dympna, you should stay with me in Omagh.' I did not want to be sucked back into life in Omagh. I wanted to be in Belfast; it was the right place for me at that time and I was going to be there. So I returned to Belfast where I had only myself to manage, where I could be to some extent free of the family and the ghosts of the family, and of Mummy going over and over the sorrows of the past as she was sure to do. I had to do this to survive although it meant that Mummy had to bear her troubles alone.

    The old life was resumed. I stayed in Belfast during the week and came back to Omagh at the weekends. All the while I was still trying to regain my old fluency in the spoken word. With people I knew and in familiar situations I could cope easily but other times and in other places my speech often failed. I would be left standing, trying to catch the word I needed in time and failing. This continually humiliated and embarrassed me. Here and there in my daily rounds my reading problem also came to the surface, both in practical situations and in my own mind. One thing which continually made me feel inadequate was the people in banks, building societies and post offices who marked the form X where I was to sign my name. I felt that my reading problem was then public knowledge, universally known. It was total humiliation for me and I felt annoyed at being stigmatised as a bad reader. I had grown up with this feeling and in primary school reading aloud in class had always been a time of trial.

Omagh Convent primary school had classes split into top and bottom grades. There was nothing to distinguish us outwardly but we all knew ourselves. I always found myself in the bottom grade but Kate, my big sister, idol and competitor, was always in the top grade. Kate passed her eleven-plus and it was felt that I too could pass my eleven-plus and so when Primary Six arrived, I found myself in Mrs Grogan's class.

Mrs Grogan was neat, precise, and business-like and I was in her net and soon to be demolished. One day she set us an essay. I put myself to the task, did what I could to the best of my ability and without any help. Daddy and Mummy could not help and Kate was too busy with her own work to oblige. When I had finished it, I did not think that it was a good essay but it was my best shot. Two days later, Mrs Grogan read out my essay to the whole class of twenty eight pupils. She read it out in a halting, stumbling manner and took it to pieces line by line, the writing, the grammar but most of all the spelling. When she had finished with it she crumpled up the page and placed it on my desk. Soon after I was demoted to Sister Mary's class. I did not tell my parents and as they never enquired much about how I was getting on at school it was easy for me to avoid the subject. I was glad to escape the tyrannies of Mrs Grogan's empire. In Sister Mary's class I gained one lasting benefit – I met Theresa McGinn.

Theresa became a close friend of mine and has remained so ever since. She was the tallest girl in the class and I was one of the smallest. She was also a great reader and there I had my problems. Theresa was a great fan of 'Biggles' books and when it came to sewing lesson she popped a Biggles book on her lap and got on with her reading while I got on with our sewing. For Theresa reading was an enjoyable pastime whereas for me it was a continuous struggle, a task, hard work. Yet through primary and then grammar school I pushed back the boundaries of my disability enough to serve my educational needs.

Six

Vincent

Conversation – that was no problem – it always came very easily to me. Each year a feis was held in the town hall and it was there that I began competing in the verse-speaking category when I was eleven. The feis was an event with a character all of its own. Every May time saw crowds of young ones, mostly six-year-olds, swarming around the doors of the town hall and down the steps onto the street. Every one of them – and their mothers – believed that they were medal-winning material and about to have this confirmed by success in their chosen category of performance. There was always a lot of bad feeling about the adjudicators who either 'knew nothing' or had their favourites or 'could neither hear nor see.' Later mothers and wee ones would return home cradling either a medal or a grudge.

The adjudicators had an impossible task on their hands, especially those who had to listen to fifty-four competitors reciting the three verses of 'My Cat Daisy.' How could any of them possibly separate a winner, remember the first while listening to the last, remember any of them at all! Outside adjudicators were appointed, wherever they could be found, but the problem remained and the struggle continued.

For several years I was among the prize-winners, although I never reached the high standards of Carol Conway. You name it, Carol Conway won it: singing, dancing, verse-speaking, wielding the bow in the traditional style or tinkling the ivories in a classical piece.

Carol was snatching firsts for medals and cups all over the place and it went on from year to year. She was a menace. We set up an anti Carol Conway Fan Club. Every morning we discussed tactics at the bus stop, on the bus and at school. Nothing we tried ever worked – Carol kept on winning everything and went on and on to greater heights.

When I was sixteen, I entered for the drama competition at the feis. In this I had to be Joan of Arc and deliver a speech. To my utter delight I won the competition and was presented with a cup for the best young actress. Wining was ecstasy and did wonders for my self-esteem. I now could compete and hold my own against all comers. I had arrived; the road was open for me; all success was possible and the world was mine.

In the middle of Omagh stands the Royal Arms Hotel and it was here that the dances were held every Saturday night. The Royal Arms became the Mecca for all the young people of the area. At this time the show band scene was at its height and many great bands like The Royal Show band, The Clipper Carlton, Joe Dolan and Big Tom and the Mainliners made regular appearances there. In the fashion of the time, the boys gathered in knots and clusters around the door and down along the side of the dance floor and we girls clustered at the far end and along the far wall, leaving a great expanse of empty floor between the sexes. When a dance was announced and the band struck up, a few nervous fellows moved forward slowly, hands in pockets, across towards us. They never made it because as soon as they made their move a stampede from behind swept them aside before they could reach their targets.

There was varied style of asking girls to dance.

'Do you want a dance?'

'Are you dancing?'

Then there were those who just grabbed a girl and pulled her onto the dance floor before she had a chance to refuse. It was a cross between a cattle stampede and a football match, and the good-looking girls were the footballs. Some girls were good lookers, some were good dancers and some were both; I was neither.

One night when the dancing started and I was not asked out I settled down to a consolation smoke.

Then, on one such night, I heard a voice.

'Would you like to dance?'

I looked up and before me stood a gorgeous young man. He looked debonair, like James Bond but smaller.

'Yes.' I said, flustered.

We took to the floor and I danced as well as I could with my stubbed cigarette in my hand. I danced that dance and the ones that followed with my new acquaintance, whose name, I discovered was Vincent. My sister Kate, who was at the dance as well, was up to a spot of matchmaking, unknown to me at the time of course. Her boyfriend and Vincent were pals at Queen's University and she had been planning to engineer a meeting but chance had intervened first. When the dance ended at about two o'clock Vincent walked me home, which was only about five minutes from the Royal Arms Hotel. It was a lovely August night, stars in the sky, stars in my eyes and a handsome and intelligent gentleman walking with me and holding my hand. I felt like a princess. I had fallen in love for the first time.

When he returned to Queen's and I was a student at Omagh Technical College doing a pre-nursing course we sent letters to each other every week. It was lovely to read and re-read Vincent's letters but somehow they were never quite up to my expectations. They were clear, precise, matter of fact but not personal enough, not romantic enough, had not enough of me or him in them. I did not realise at the time what a reserved man Vincent was, and that it was a family trait you did not pour out your feelings about yourself or others – words were for using with restraint. As his mother, God rest her, used to say, 'If you haven't something good to say, say nothing.'

During this period the Civil Rights movement had begun their campaign and Vincent and myself got involved in the marches. It seemed to us then that things were on the mend and that this was part of the process. When later I went to the Royal Victoria Hospital I saw what a bomb can do to a human body. I saw soldiers with arms and legs blown off, others with plastic tubes where their intestines had been but like so many others, I little dreamed that it would all turn out as it did. Later I joined the Peace Movement and went on their marches.

For years Vincent and I went out together and after that time he was keen to get settled down – but I was not at all interested. Settling down was not on my agenda; not even on the horizon of my vision. I was heading for Belfast and a nursing job in the Royal Victoria Hospital the following September. I wanted to be footloose and fancy free. So we parted but not in anger. We remained good friends and Vincent always remained his helpful and considerate self. My mother could not understand my attitude. She had been a constant admirer of Vincent from the beginning and never tired of telling me what a good catch he was, how good and kind and reliable he was, how considerate he was to everyone. 'Why don't you marry him?' Mother would constantly ask. 'l don't love him, Mummy,' was my constant reply and I would put my hand on her shoulder as a kind of defence against her insistence. She never did understand.

After the death of Rosaleen I found life difficult. I needed friends, a friend to cry with. My then boyfriend was not very supportive. One day I wandered into the living-room in Ireton Street and there was Vincent. I walked over to him, buried my face in his chest and cried. He put his arms around me and kissed me warmly, as warmly as he had ever done, and in that instant I saw him as others saw him, as Mummy saw him. I recalled in my mind some of the countless ways he had befriended me, never asking for anything in return. Vincent was the one who had always been there when I needed a friend – a rare treasure. For once my head and my heart were in agreement. Vincent was ready to restart our previous relationship. I had been given one more chance and I knew that I had to get things right this time. How I must have hurt him when I rejected him! Now he seemed to me to be my guardian angel. I could not mess things up again. Vincent could not take being hurt again. I was resolved – I would get things right this time round.

In the summer of 1980, when I was twenty six years old, we got married in Drumragh Parish Church and had the reception in the Royal Arms Hotel, where Vincent had disrupted my comforting smoke ten years previously. Many momentous days had passed in those ten years but my marriage day was the best day's work of those ten years and all the twenty-six years as well.

When Vincent rose to speak after the meal, he finished by explaining to our guests that we had just had our first argument and that I had won.

On hearing this everyone paid attention. Vincent then announced that his newly-wedded wife, contrary to all tradition and convention, was going to address the guests. They say that the wedding day is the bride's day, so I thought it only proper that I should have my say. Would I struggle over the words, I didn't even care, it was our day.

For the next five or six minutes I welcomed the guests and thanked them for coming and celebrating our great day with us.

They listened to me with great attention and clapped heartily when at the finish.

Soon afterwards we began to live our married life together in the friendly old house in Ireton Street.

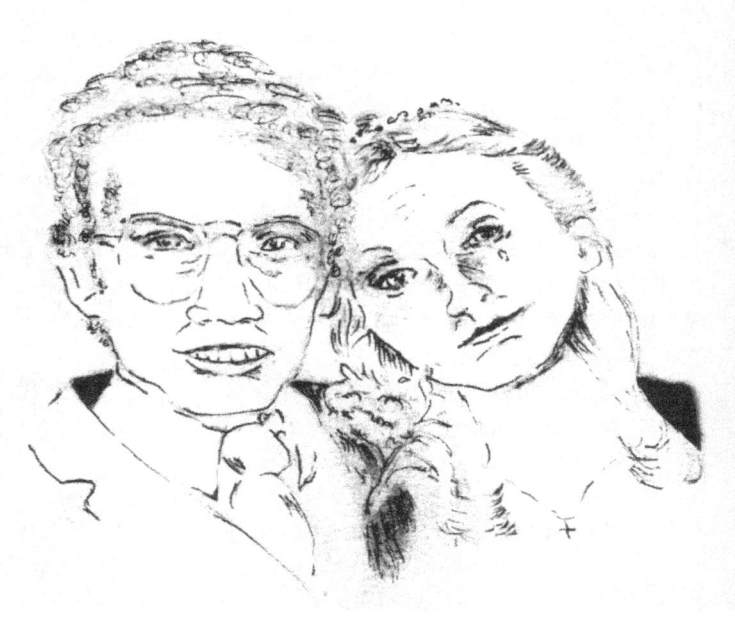

The best day's work of those ten years

After university Vincent began his career working as an electrical engineer with the Electricity Board but had not found this work very fulfilling. He wanted a role which was more people-centred and had his heart on a job in community development. He did a two-year course at the polytechnic and after qualifying he got a post in the Community Services Department of Lisburn Borough Council. With this job came a move for us from the house in Ireton Street to a spanking-new white semi-detached house in a new housing estate in Lisburn.

It was quite a wrench for us to leave Ireton Street. The old house had many happy memories for us. It was a three-storey terrace house, old, perhaps a hundred years old and was situated in the university area of the city. While Vincent owned it, it had been host to a number of university students, friends, and cousins, people from his work place and passers by or visitors who had made a short stay under its roof. It carried with it many good memories of events, get-togethers and people, and of Christmas parties when certain residents got a brush, a Brillo pad, a mop, or a dishcloth wrapped in Christmas paper to remind them that the old place needed some attention. No one ever acted on the hint. The house was nevertheless old and damp, and living in it entailed a lot of stair climbing – so move we did.

While Vincent busied himself at his new work, looking after rent, rates, mortgages, electricity and gas bills and spoiling me in the process, I decided to do a course in 'Drama and Related studies' and who was the lecturer but my old friend John! After his visit to Omagh to see me he had kept in regular touch. He was continually concerned for me and wanted to know how I was coping. When I returned to Belfast, he called on me regularly and on such occasions I carefully avoided talking about the accident. I did not want to upset him. The old relationship was gone, if it ever existed and now the only common bond between us was the accident. He had disposed of his walking stick and as I mentioned earlier, was driving a car again and had returned to his old job at the polytechnic. His life had returned to normal or nearly so and he was intending to get married.

He wanted me to meet Ann and I had a feeling that in some way he wanted my approval. So the plan was agreed and John took me in his car to see his girlfriend Ann who lived somewhere on the Lisburn Road. It seemed very strange that here was I still very interested in John but not as marriage material and here was John introducing me to Ann and wanting me to commend his choice. Ann shared a second-floor flat with another girl and there we were introduced in a room that was most noticeable for the number of sewing-machines that were scattered all over the place. Ann struck me as a pleasant and sincere person and as John drove me home I told him so; he seemed pleased to hear it. Later they married and had a family of three.

It was John who had suggested to me that I take up the course and that is how I found myself a student again but the experience was not as before; the magic was gone. Time had slipped on. Where were my old friends? In jobs, marking out their careers, earning good money. The drama course was interesting and enjoyable but it had not the meaning of the one before: that had a purpose and an end-product that was my ambition. The students working on this course had come from councils, health boards, community service, all working people, and then there was me, the woman who did not work for a living but did voluntary work for the NSPCC and the Simon Community.

One afternoon we were training in the gym. The exercise was meant to teach us the skills of communication, learning to trust and be at ease in the company of others. Suddenly out of the blue a student suggested we kiss the person to whom we were talking. Whether the proposal was meant to embarrass someone or out of self-interest I don't know but as soon as it was made, John climbed up a pole and stayed planted until the kissing game was finished. We sat down and discussed together what the game revealed about attitudes and behaviour and when it came to John's turn to comment he said he did not want to kiss anyone in the group.

John's reaction surprised me greatly. It seemed so untypical of him. He had been a very outgoing person before and this mechanical peck on the cheek business would have been merely a feather in the wind once but now it put him to flight. I could not help thinking that it was my presence there that had bought about this unexpected reaction. Was he thinking of that wet February night at the bend of the road? I don't know. At the end of the course we were all successful and departed with a certificate. By this time, in late autumn of 1982, I was expecting my first child.

Seven

Birth and Death

I remember first seeing a scan of this human being with legs and arms moving inside me. It was an incredible sight full of wonder, mystery, majesty, a spectacular miraculous happening within me. I was a house and home, love, care and carriage to this little one, this new human being. I was dumbfounded, even shocked, by this new experience and the wholeness of my new responsibilities. Now everything depended on me. Could I cope, was I up to the task, would I be successful to the end? Yet despite the questions, my feelings were always positive. I will succeed; we will succeed' a miracle is taking place – we are becoming parents. This little one is our destiny to love and cherish, to care for all the days of our lives: with us our child will grow and develop. succeed, reach full potential. In all the days of expecting that followed feelings of wonder, excitement and some unease remained with me and all the while I myself had become and was becoming a new person.

As the time of my delivery approached I became huge and felt embarrassed by my appearance. We went to the Royal Maternity Hospital for the birth and though husbands should not be there at a forceps delivery I insisted that Vincent was present. I held on to his hand through all the labour. It was an exciting time with a new feel of power and responsibility and on the 13th March 1983 I gave birth to a baby boy weighing 9lb 12oz. Mothers always remember the weight of their babies! I had an almighty pride in myself after delivering the big son and heir to the family fortune and I waited patiently to be showered with flowers. It had been no easy task, accident and all, and I deserved to be treated royally but in this my poor man was a disaster. He did manage to send me a postcard which I received after I returned home. That Vincent had to go to work, manage the house, do his shopping, cook for himself (if he did) visit me each day, and be with me while I was giving birth, did not seem enough of an understanding of a woman's world.

My mother phoned the hospital to see how I was getting on. I was a mother now; I had gone through the pain of giving birth; I had been successful in a great event and when it was over I felt a great sense of joy, especially when I looked at this fine big baby. I thought Mummy had always been too negative whenever she talked to us about our coming into the world. Those were the thoughts that turned in my head as I spoke to her on the phone that evening. I cannot remember what I said but it must have been quite sharp. She promised to come up and visit us in Lisburn on the following Friday when I would be out of hospital but that was not to be.

On the following Friday she took ill and was taken to hospital in Omagh, and on the Saturday morning we gathered up our things and set off there. When we arrived we discovered that mother was in the Intensive Care Unit and we were not allowed to enter. We sat there for two hours, me attending the baby and Vincent trying to pass the time. It was then that the doctor came out to tell me that my mother was dead. There had been no chance to say 'l love you' to say a word of thanks, to say a word at all.

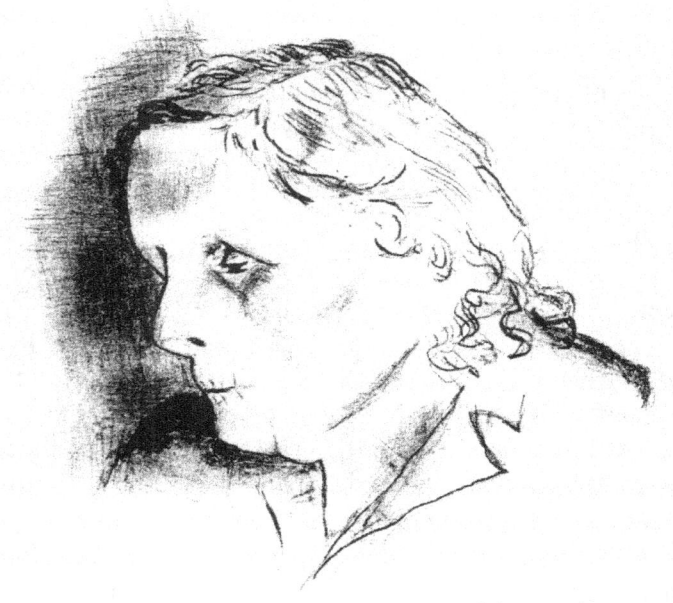

My mother

Kate had married and she too had a young baby, only two months old. There we were, the two of us, in Mummy's house with our babies on our knees while the house filled up with people coming to the wake.

Next day we toasted ourselves in front of the gas-cooker to kill the cold of March. We were about to set out for the great cathedral-sized Church of the Sacred Heart in Omagh. The splendid church with its lofty roof, its ornate high altar and its glorious many-storied stained glass window above would make a striking setting for any funeral but those who had come to pay a last tribute seemed small and sparse in the great space. Mummy was never an outgoing person, never had a wide circle of friends, her friends were her family and a few others. She had never been a goer, an organiser, and especially after the death of Rosaleen, these traits in her became more pronounced. In her last years she became a lonely woman living alone in her house, drifting from day to day. It seemed as if she had died a long time before her funeral.

It was Kate who had been head of the family long before Mummy's end. Kate was smart, bustling, ambitious, articulate. Mother and daughter –same nature, same nurture – so different, so differing. Mother did settle her affairs. She left the house to Pat, the glassware to Kate and the family portraits to me. She had a good collection of original portraits once but over the years had given them away one by one until there were only a few left. When the funeral was over and family affairs settled we went back to our own places and took up life where we had left off.

After the move from the old house, with its damp, its stairs, its cramped surroundings a move to a new white semi-detached house in Lisburn seemed a move for the better but it turned out to be far different. All my life I had been surrounded by people I did not know and did not have the opportunity to get to know. I began to feel the isolation, the 'new suburb blues' that are said to affect new mothers and wives. Even after the arrival of Paul, the feeling remained. The old places with their comings and goings of people, the get-togethers, their memories, good and bad, but mostly good, took on a fresh gloss for me now. It was the time of the Anglo-Irish Agreement and there was a great resentment among the Unionist people against it, and though the Troubles had never worried us in the old places, they now seemed to be a constant threat. So when the time came to leave I did so without regret or any feeling for the new white semi-detached house in the new estate.

We had kept in regular touch with friends in Omagh and most weekends saw us speeding down the M1 with Paul well secured in his safety seat in the back. On one occasion he gave us an almighty fright. We had travelled about five miles from home when I looked behind me to see how he was.'Stop, stop, stop!' I cried out. Vincent managed to pull over and stop without causing an accident. 'What's wrong?' he asked, looking into the back seat. The carry cot was there all right but there was no Paul. Vincent had forgotten him, I had forgotten him, we had forgotten him. We found a turning point and raced back. He was probably bawling and the neighbours out sounding an alert. We arrived. There was no one about, no one in the gardens, no one looking out their windows. We slowed to a normal approaching speed and entered the driveway quietly, sedately. He was still sound asleep in his cot, not a feather astray on him. We were so grateful and, needless to say, we never forgot him again.

We still kept in touch with John and his family and visited several times a year. We never talked about the bond that was keeping us together: for me it was that terrible night of the accident. We would talk about everything except the accident. In any case the children were always present. John had counselling after the accident but even if I had been offered counselling I was having none of it. I was strong and I did not need to stoop to that. I did not want to discuss the results of the accident nor allow them into my life. I remember once when Kate was home from England she suggested that I would be entitled to a Disability Card. I remember that I was ironing at the time. I put down the iron, looked at her furiously and said, 'No, No!' I wanted none of that – no disability, no counselling. I would cope by myself, manage by myself. I was strong; I could 'cut it.'

Eight

E For Epilepsy

We returned to Omagh where Vincent had secured a post with Omagh District Council. We first lived in a cottage in Gortin in the heart of the country. Two years after the birth of Paul, Catherine arrived, and two years after that came Una. Both were born in Omagh Maternity Hospital which is now unfortunately closed, so mothers have to travel to another county to have their babies delivered.

With three small children to attend to I was fully occupied and had little time to foster my continuing education needs but I did manage to join the literacy group at Omagh College of Further Education. When Paul was three years old I got involved in the setting up of a parents and toddlers group. I found this very satisfying as it introduced me to many young families in the area as well as being very worthwhile in its own right. I continued to be involved with the parents' group until Una was eight years old.

It was when the morning rush to school was over, the dishes washed, the tidying up done and the house quiet that I began to reassess my future. I wanted to acquire a skill that would lead to a full-time paid post in Omagh. I set my heart on acquiring a qualification in a child care. I had already gone through a quite extensive series of courses in my re-education after the accident. I had been with Miss Keys for speech therapy, the adult literacy programme in Belfast, to Miss Hill, a foundation course in pre-school study, a pre-school playgroup course and the course in drama and related studies conducted by John. Now I wanted to pit myself against a GCSE syllabus and for this I chose Child Psychology. This course demanded a lot of work and effort on my part. After studying a topic I was set to write the first draft of an essay on it. I then took this to my tutor, who worked through it with me and then we worked through it again and produced a final essay.

I diligently learned key words and topics in preparation for the coming examination. This was fine as far as it went but the examination with the pressure of a set time to complete the paper and having to recall everything instantly was a different thing. When I sat down in the gymnasium of the college trying to read the questions I had to answer, I did not understand some of them and others I did not read correctly. The pressure to perform under strict limits was pressing down on me but I did give it my full stroke. When I looked at my finished paper I found it was littered with spelling mistakes and the language was disjointed. At the end of the paper I wrote, 'Thank you for reading this.' John had sent me a card wishing me well in the examination. The results would come in August. Oh God!

On the day when the exam results were due, we had planned to take a short holiday in Rossnowlagh in Donegal. The morning was very crowded making preparations for this stay, washing, sorting, packing, quelling arguing children – at least there was no danger of leaving any of them behind! A milkman to be informed, a dog and cat to be resettled. All morning I had been rushing around, doing a dozen different tasks at once and hoping to squeeze in enough time to call at the college and collect my results. We managed it and I stepped forward to find out how I had done. An E – so much work; so little return I was very depressed.

We headed off to Rossnowlagh with Vincent driving, me beside him and the tug-of-war team of three in the back. A little way out we re-arranged the cargo, Vincent still driving, Paul beside him and me a peace line in the back. We arrived safe and sound at Rossnowlagh with its expansive beach. The day was cloudy and grey. By chance John's two teenage sons, Jerry and Edward, were there with their wet suits and surf boards. I passed them in the deep water. 'This is a great place to surf.' Said Jerry as he skimmed past on his board. 'Have a good day,' I replied as I too plunged into the water and did a few back strokes. I attempted to stand up and found myself out of my depth. Torrents of water rolled over me. I was being swept away. 'What am I going to do?' I thought. 'Be calm. Be calm.' There were people around. Another torrent of water passed over me. I was further out form the beach now. I was being swept out – drowning. 'Help, help, help!' I screamed. No one came to rescue me.

With my life in my hands I changed course and struggled frantically towards the beach. I don't know how I managed it but I got there. The ground was firm beneath my feet and I was walking from the water. 'Did you hear someone shouting for help, Mummy?' Una asked. She was playing at the water's edge. 'That was me,' I said shaking with exhaustion and shock. 'I nearly drowned.' Una put her little arms around my waist and started to cry. We had planned to stay there two or three days and Kate, who was home from England at the time, joined us. We were staying just outside Rossnowlagh and it was here that I had another epileptic fit the night after my near drowning.

An epileptic fit is a very frightening experience for the sufferer and for anyone witnessing it. When I am having a fit, so I've been told, my whole body goes rigid, I clench my teeth and flail about me. There is a danger that I could bite my tongue or injure myself as I try to catch my breath, drawing in air in great distressed gulps through my mouth and nose. Most embarrassing of all, I sometimes wet the bed. When Vincent witnessed me having a fit for the first time he thought I was dying. This was seven years after the accident and the medical explanation appears to be that the scar tissue on any wound is not the same as the original tissue. The fit occurs when the brain is short-circuited and the whole system is thrown into a state of extreme panic. Then follows a wild struggle to survive, to get back on course, to function normally. When the fit is over, there is a period of extreme exhaustion which takes a whole day or more to overcome.

When we got back from holiday a great feeling of defeat and depression came over me. I wanted to cry and cry and cry but when the children were present I hid my feelings and kept them to myself. I put on a bright and cheerful face and pretended that everything was rosy. As soon as the children went to bed my defences broke and I cried and cried and cried. Vincent kept asking, 'Whatever is the matter with you?'

'I don't know,' I would say. 'I know it's something to do with the accident. I must go to the doctor. I can't go on like this.'

When I met my doctor he promised to get me some help and arranged an appointment with a clinical psychologist. I was put on a waiting list and a month later, two months later, I had no word and was still waiting.

Every year Dr Johnson, the neurosurgeon at the Royal Victoria Hospital, visits the local hospital to see former patients. I saw him in June, by which time I had been waiting ten months for the appointment with the clinical psychologist. I tried not to cry but, as I began to pour out my troubles, my tears began to flow in front of this strong and eminent neurosurgeon. 'I'm good for nothing,' I whimpered. 'I am a failure and I cannot help myself.'

I looked at him, surprised. He was not condescending, not full of pity for me. He seemed to be speaking the bare truth. I looked at him, so big and important, a distinguished man at the top of his profession. 'Sometimes I feel the same as yourself, Dympna – yes, we all have to live with failure,' he said. My brown mascara was running all over my face and I had no tissue.

'How can you say that? I asked, 'You are at the top your profession.' I got up and got myself a tissue.

'Yes I am quite good at my work,' the doctor said. 'But when I am at home I feel depressed sometimes.'

This is getting too personal, I thought. Before, he was the medical expert whom I saw once a year; I had not seen his human side. Now, he was taking down the barriers and revealing himself to a mere patient as just another patient, subject to pain.

'But I need someone to help me, Doctor,' and I told him of the appointment that never was.

'I won't promise anything,' he said but I'll see what I can do.

By now my entire make up was off and as I left the surgery my tear-stained face plainly told my state. It seemed to me that everyone was looking at me but I did not care.

Nine

Facing it

We visited John's family again around the New Year of 1994. We were all staying over for the night and I intended to talk to John alone about what had happened nearly twenty years before. When I had first suffered an epileptic fit, my doctor had given me strict instructions on how to manage my problem: never get overtired; always make sure you get a good night's sleep, no alcohol, no cigarettes, no drugs whatsoever.

That was the sentence but it was not such a hard lifestyle to follow. I was a married woman with a good husband, a comfortable home and three lovely children. If this had happened when I was a teenager, then things might have been much harder to manage; with no late dances or parties, the doctor's guidelines would have checked and confined me at every bend. I would have been like Cinderella with no Fairy Godmother. Even in my settled days there were occasions, and this was one of them, when I needed to break doctor's orders. I stayed on. I wanted to talk to John alone but my concentration was slipping. The conversation was not going my way; yet I was determined to say my piece.

'Have you ever given a thought for what the accident has done to me?'

'What, Dympna? What do you mean?'

'Have you ever given a thought for what the accident has done to me?' I repeated.

John put down his glass of red wine. His brown-grey hair was receding and cut very short. He sat by the fire in the front room of their bungalow. I sat upright on the sofa, looking him straight in the eye. His eyes were sad and he looked concerned.

'Would you like some wine?' he asked.

'I can't take any alcohol because of my fits, John!' I angrily replied. He looked shocked.

'When did this happen?'

'Seven years after the accident and it's because of the accident that I have them.'

'You never told me.'

'I did not want to hurt your feelings,' I said, 'and besides, I thought that it was completely my fault.'

'I thought that you were through all your feelings on the accident,' said John. 'You never told me about them.'

'How could l?' I asked, 'They were all negative. I will never have a real qualification because I don't have the wherewithal to express myself.'

John moved over to sit beside me on the sofa. I could feel the tears coming but I did not want to cry. I wanted to be a strong lady who was giving him information about Dympna: about Dympna who would never be the same again because of the accident, about a Dympna who had been kept from him, for his sake.

'I will never have a career.' I said coldly.

John never spoke a single word.

My tears began to flow thick and fast. John's head was bent and his shoulders stooped. For the first time in my life I let him see me cry. I was falling asunder. My speech became worse and worse; I needed to go to bed. I got up to go. We did not touch. He now began to realise a part of me that had been kept hidden for years and the reality of what had happened on that terrible night.

When I asked to have an appointment with a clinical psychologist I was told that I might have to wait some time. That sometime was a year and a half and by then I had most of my crying done. Meanwhile the dismal examination result, the near-drowning, the epileptic fits had all come together, forming a catalyst to bring about the changes within me.

Gradually I began to discard the 'I'll be all right tomorrow' belief, to acknowledge that something permanent had happened which would be with me today, tomorrow and all the tomorrows.

I began to form a perspective of the accident. No longer did I see myself responsible for it but rather the victim. In my mind John had become the object of my rage and the more I blamed him the more my hostility towards him grew and festered within me. In my view he had escaped, got away scot-free. He had picked up his life and career again untouched, probably never gave the accident a thought now in his daily rounds. For me, even twenty years later, it remained a continuous net around me, tripping me up, entangling me, and thwarting my every effort to throw it off. Though it was true that I had done most of my crying before the first meeting with the clinical psychologist I cried for most of the first session. In the second session I tried to explain the events in my life that had brought me to seek her help. In the third session she began to set out guidelines for me to follow, explaining to me that for some people it is impossible to talk about unfortunate events in their lives. She advised me to pick three friends who I knew and trusted and talk over the accident and its consequences with them. I was taken quite aback with this advice. I had come to this professional seeking help and had felt forgotten for a year and a half when the help did not come. I felt that the clinical psychologist was passing the problem back to me and my friends to solve. It seemed that I had come on a long journey only to arrive back at the point of departure – a physician saying; 'Patient cure thyself.'

Do I know what I want to say to my friends? Do I want to unload my problems onto them? Do I want to reveal that much of myself to them? Do I have three friends that I trust enough to go down this road with them? All these questions were playing on my mind but I decided to give it a try so I picked three friends, Theresa, my old school friend, and Mary and Margaret, friends from Belfast days. They all knew about my accident of course, and since it had happened all that time ago they had seen me marry, raise my children and take an active part in the life in the community. As far as they were aware from the outside I had coped fully with the accident and had fully recovered. Now I was coming to them saying that this was not so, that they had been deceived by appearances and that I was confiding in them because I needed their help to deal with problems which they had believed had been buried a long time ago. I had always been a communicator but now I vowed to be a listener. That was the task before me and how I saw it.

I wore my heart upon my sleeve, talked things out with Teresa, talked things out with Mary. I listened to their responses and it helped. Another time I would talk to Margaret too. It dawned on me slowly that tomorrow would not be better than today, nor any other day for the rest of my life.

At this time we were planning to go to the USA for a holiday. Kate drove us down to Dublin and on the way Una was sick three times. We began to doubt the wisdom of travelling on such a long journey, to the USA and then across it, with three small children, aged ten, eight and six, and of course Una's doll, Baby Born, had to be taken too as there would have been holy uproar if it had been left behind.

Things turned out better than we could have expected. We crossed the Atlantic, crossed the American continent and although Una had been sick three times on the way from Omagh to Dublin Airport she was not sick once the whole way across America. Most people have relatives in America and we were no exception. We went to visit my Aunt Elizabeth in New York. She is an eighty-three year old Yankee grandmother, active and hustling, interested and interesting and very well organised. She arranged for her sons and daughters to show us around the sights of New York. It was late July, the huge city was like a furnace and the Brogans panted their way through downtown New York in a lather of sweat. We had to take the children with us. They were crying and complaining most of the time because of the heat but we held on tightly to each other and we arrived back at Elizabeth's house with no one missing.

A shining house and food on the table awaited us. Thanks to wee Una, Baby Born arrived back safely too. For the week we were there we were treated like royalty. Next door, unknown to Elizabeth, lived the McCullagh family, who originated from Plumbridge and who were, we discovered, second cousins of Vincent's.

After leaving Elizabeth we flew off to the Pacific Coast and San Francisco with two big suitcases, three small children and Una's inseparable doll. In San Francisco we walked or used public transport wherever we went but soon became aware that our mode of transport was out of fashion and that anyone who was anyone was driving around in an air-conditioned car. Walking and public transport were for poor blacks and poor whites. Amid the razzmatazz of this fresh glittering city I couldn't avoid noticing the grinding poverty of the unsuccessful who advertised their plight with placards saying 'l need work. I have no money' and offering their labour to anyone who cared to buy it but at miserable rates of pay.

After San Francisco we hired a light blue, air-conditioned car and set off to Oregon, a journey of approximately 400 miles and at two o' clock in the morning we reached our destination. There before us was Margaret, with outstretched arms ready to greet us. We piled out of the car, all five of us like prisoners set free after the confinement of the long hot journey. We had come all this way to make contact again with Margaret and her husband, Jamie.

Margaret was originally Swiss. She was a teacher by profession but had come to Belfast as a VSO and worked in community care in the Shankhill area of the city. There she met her husband Jamie form Oregon who was likewise a community care worker in the Falls Road area. It was the time of the Vietnam War and Jamie was in Belfast doing community care to avoid being sent to Vietnam to fight in a faraway war.

They both attended weekend course in drama and it was there that I came to know them. After they married and settled down in Oregon, Jamie's home state, we kept in touch.

They were coordinators of a camp, a holiday reflection-community centre. People came here to relax, to escape the pressures of modern living, and to reflect on their way of life. The camp was set in a beautiful wooded area with lots of water, sky and space. Up until now in all our journeys about America we were thinking about the safety of the children, counting, collecting, recollecting and hanging on to them. But here we all relaxed and the children enjoyed the freedom and the open spaces like uncaged birds.

While we were there a group of native American children were in residence. They had come to learn the old forgotten skills of their forefathers: carving, leather work, painting.

There is an ever-present danger that the old Indian customs and skills could be wiped away entirely. The language remains in the names of rivers, lakes, hills, place names and words that have passed into English. Yet it must be humiliating that the once free proud Native American has come down to this, to have to relearn their own old ways at the feet of their conqueror.

One night a group of us went out with Jamie and Margaret to a hill outside the camp to observe a night sky spectacle. From the hill we could observe a meteor shower. Suddenly a shower of stars came rushing down from the sky and then vanished completely. This process happened again and again and for the next half hour we watched until even this spectacular night sky event began to lose its magic. By the end of the evening I had seen enough to last me a life time.

Margaret was a busy, hustling type of woman and I was waiting my turn to snatch an opportunity to talk to her about my own situation, about how the accident had affected me and how it was affecting me at the present time. I wanted to talk to her alone without the botheration of children or adults. It now seems a very long way and an expensive way to have come to chat to one person alone. Northern Ireland is a very small place, and I wanted to talk to someone that I trusted and to know that whatever was said or whatever names were spoken that I could feel assured that all I said remained sealed. There was an ocean and a continent between and, besides, I trusted Margaret.

She talked and discussed my story and she commented and questioned, teasing matters out and giving me her opinions in her forthright way.

'Did you talk to John about how you feel?'

'I tried to but he avoided it.'

'You need to tell him exactly how you feel,' she said firmly, 'without letting him interrupt.'

'Yes.' I said as I looked into her blue green eyes.

I was always passive with John after the accident, taking blame and responsibility upon myself, shielding him from the realities. Now I felt the need to protect myself, to assert myself, to be active in the direction of my own life. I wanted to speak to John on my own terms, in my own place and tell him exactly how I felt. Despite all my efforts and determination up until now I had always felt that I had not been a planner nor a doer in life and that that role had been imposed on me by others.

Margaret had pointed the way for me and how I should do it and I hoped I would be equal to the task.

We arrived home from the USA safe and well with the three children still in tow and Baby Born in the arms of wee Una. Kate was waiting for us at the airport and it was her birthday. Next day Vincent went off to work, the children went off to school and I went on with the housework and washed masses of clothes.

Ten

Talking to John

'Would you like to come down to my house on Wednesday' I asked John over the phone, 'about 11 o'clock?'

'Yes, Dympna,' he replied.

High noon in Brogan's kitchen.

At exactly 11 o'clock John walked up to my door.

'Where is your car? I asked immediately.

'It's at home. I got the bus down to Omagh.'

'Come in. Come in,' and I brought him in from the hall to the kitchen.

'Do you know why I asked you to come?

'Yes, I do,' he answered as he sat down on the red settee in the kitchen and I sat on the table bench near to him.

'I want to talk to you about the accident and how it has affected me twenty-one years later. Since the accident I have tried very hard to make something of myself. I cannot even get a GCSE in any subject, John.'

He was silent.

'Can you not even say to me, "I am sorry Dympna"?' I shouted. 'Everything I worked at and worked for was lost in those few seconds. My life has been wasted and the person who has been responsible for all this can't even say, "I am sorry"'. My voice began to rise again. I wanted to see him cry. He put his head down and looked at the floor.

'I am not going to feel sorry for you. I am not! I am not! You got off scot- free: I took all the baggage and the blame. Why did you not stop me going that night?'

'But you were an adult! You seemed so mature!' John finally answered as he raised his head and looked at me.

'I was a twenty year-old student. You were a thirty-year-old lecturer, a man of power. I was infatuated with your position of power, not with you, John. All my life I had tried to become someone and I was succeeding, and you swept it all away in one minute,' I cried. 'I know you have not heard much of this before but that was because I did not want to hurt your feelings.'

I got up and found myself a tissue, 'I want you to say I am sorry.'

'lf it makes things any better.. I am sorry. I am sorry for the accident,' John said. 'I thought that when I came up to your house for the first time your father would kill me for what has happened but then there was no father. Your people welcomed me and treated me with respect and courtesy, and when I saw you getting much better with your speech all the time, I thought you had fully recovered.'

'All the words I have in my vocabulary I have had to work bloody hard for, but the accident and its consequences are forever with me.'

'Yes. I know,' he said quietly, as he stared down at the floor.

'Do you not think it would have been a good idea not to allow me to get into the car that night?' I demanded. There was vengeance in my voice now.

'You made your own choice; you wanted to go with me, Dympna.'

I made no reply. A visible silence filled the kitchen. The ticking of the clock grew and grew. Finally, John said, 'You were very persuasive then, as you are now. I didn't know there was going to be an accident, Dympna, but I am sorry, sorry.'

The tears began to well up in my eyes and spill on to my cheeks. The tears I wanted to see from him did not come.

'Have you got time to eat, John?' I said, changing subject entirely as I wiped my tears away.

'Just about.'

We had something to eat and made ready to go. We stopped outside the entrance. I turned into the garage to fetch my bike and we set off on the road towards the bus station. I felt that his conversation should have taken place a lot earlier but if it had I would still be waiting for a miracle to happen, to be back where I was before the accident. You mature and develop further until the day you die and that is a fact for everyone.

On seeing me wheeling the bicycle John cheered up a bit.

'When did you start using your bicycle?' he asked.

'Oh years ago,' I smiled.

We both smiled.

'Thank you for never abandoning me after the accident; many people would.'

'Thank you for saying that, Dympna.'

We passed the sign that pointed the way to Omagh. We walked together the mile or so of the road until the bus station was in view, filling the empty spaces with neutral conversation and said our goodbyes at the bus station. The bus pulled out and he was on his way.

It was twenty-one years after the accident and John was beginning to look old. I had said what I needed to say to him, what was inside me for a long time, my speech was good. I felt that I was in control of my own life now. A weight had been lifted off me. I was free. I got on my bike and headed off home exhilarated, never touching the ground.

Now that I had my say, the searing anger in me began to subside and die. I began to feel more reconciled with my world, more at ease with myself than I had been for a very long time. It had taken me a long time to realise that all the past could not be retrieved and that the todays were the reality. Perhaps there was too much of me to leave behind but compromise and reconciliation had come and I began to look at the present and the future with a calmer satisfaction. I had a last reached a plateau of contentment which I hoped was wide enough to give me sufficient space for the rest of my life.

I remember one day when I was a nurse in the Royal walking down the Grosvenor Road with a colleague when we began to talk about a patient, a soldier who had suffered brain damage. My colleague asked me, 'How would you cope with brain damage?'

'I don't know,' I replied and that is true: we all react differently. There are many ways of dealing with loss, from meek acceptance to rebellion, from striving wholeheartedly against it, to quietly pushing back the frontiers. I had struggled relentlessly to recover my former condition – maybe too hard – but I believed and still believe that if I had not done so, then I would have remained in the wilderness where I first found myself.

My thoughts often went back to Miss Key's group therapy class. Miss Key sat at her table and we were wheeled into her room. She talked to us all through the session. No one else spoke a word. Some were unable to speak a word and for others the effort required was too great. Some were pleading for help and their eyes were their voices but others were uninterested, not involved, resigned to a life in a land of limbo – and their eyes said it too.

'No!' I kept saying to myself, 'I am never going to be one of those,' while Miss Key went on and on with our speech therapy. And my speech? My speech, the jewel of my being, is reasonable and sometimes great when I am speaking to one person. When I am speaking to several, if I had a good night's sleep the night before and if the people to whom I am speaking are interested in what I have to say, then my speech is passable. However, if the people to whom I am speaking give me the impression of not listening or are not interested, then my speech is extremely poor. If I strive to regain control, the effort only intensifies my confusion.

I still get annoyed when I don't have the right words to express what I want to say or respond to a situation as quickly as I would like. My reading and writing are poor as well. This has been a very hard thing to say because of the stigma that is still attached to people like myself who have great problems with numeracy and literacy. I have been a student of the Adult Literacy Programme for twenty-one years now. The programme itself is staffed by volunteers and enables students to cope with the language and maths skills which we all need now. The time, patience, energy and commitment of the tutors are second to none. This book would not have been written nor would it have been possible for me to do the courses I have done without the back-up of the tutors. The literacy course has helped me to live a more fulfilled life and has been a life line to me.

Eleven

Now

And what am I now? I am a wife and mother with a head injury. I am the woman who started the Parent and Toddler Group in Omagh, an organisation which has given great benefit and enjoyment to its members and from which I have now retired. I have recently joined Headway, a support group for brain-injured people and their families. Headway organises talks by medical experts and I am very excited about its work and the benefits and understanding it can bring.

Meanwhile I am a full time housewife doing a multitude of tasks: washing, cleaning, brushing, sewing, ironing, folding, sorting, arranging, packing, dusting, decorating, soothing, scolding, enticing, encouraging, wheedling, humouring, praising, roasting, basting, carving, ladling, shopping, banking, budgeting, bargaining, judging, jurying, coaxing, bribing, bullying, investigating, baking, boiling, doctoring, dispensing, and forgetting – a woman's work is never done! It all adds up to an epic achievement; and then there's looking after myself.

Patrick Kavanagh, the Monaghan small farmer turned poet, says much the same thing in one of his poems. He looks at a man with his harrow and horse team sowing a field of corn. In the mind of the poet this ordinary farm task becomes mystical and elemental, an almost religious event. It is an act of faith in the soil and in God the Creator and the sower himself. The seed is the harvest that will be and the sower is the key participant in a wondrous and epic event.

TO THE MAN AFTER THE HARROW

> Now leave the check-reins slack,
> The seed is flying far today -
> The seed like stars against the black
> Eternity of April clay.
>
> This seed is potent as the seed
> Of knowledge in the Hebrew Book,
> So drive your horses in the creed
> Of God the Father as a stook.
>
> Forget the men on Brady's Hill.
> Forget what Brady's boy may say.
> For destiny will not fulfil
> Unless you let the harrow play.
>
> Forget the worm's opinion too
> Of hooves and pointed harrow-pins,
> For you are driving your horses through
> The mist where Genesis begins.

(Reproduced by kind permission of the trustees of the estate of Patrick Kavanagh)

Some say that managing a house and a home and raising a family successfully is the peak of all achievement and I am ready to agree. The only problem is that one never knows when the task is finished and the recognition can be claimed. So far I am very happy and have had great satisfaction and much joy from the task and I pray that it continues so.

For several years I have been re-visiting an old haunt, the annual May Feis in the town hall. The old routine is still the same, crowds of young ones, especially four, five, six and seven year-olds with angel faces and hearts full of the hope of going home with a medal or even a cup. The mothers too are there, confirming the faith of the young ones. The only difference is that a generation has passed and the old town hall looks more than ever in need of a heart and lungs transplant.

Catherine has entered for the Feis for several years and has won a number of awards. At the last Feis we attended Una had made a big effort on her recitation event and was hopeful but there were scores of other competitors. When the results were announced Una had gained a joint second – out of so many! Catherine did not get a mention, not even a recommendation. I looked at Catherine; she seemed uncomfortable. She had put a great effort into the work over several weeks.

'Are you disappointed?' I asked.

'No, not really,' she replied, 'I'm just glad wee Una won something.' I was relieved and proud of her. Una came down from the stage clutching her medal in her hand and held it out for us to see. She was purring with pleasure. We set off for home together, cradling a medal and happiness. Una was already making plans to ambush Dad with the good news as soon as he stepped over the threshold.

Yes, things are improving.

Paul had been the first to dip his toe in the waters of the feis, but he found them cold and uninviting. For him the world of the sciences and particularly the call of computers was more attractive and he took to the new technologies with the active support of his dad. Now he speaks the strange language of CAD, ROM, RAM and eats his food thinking of bytes and megabytes. It's very boring – and he'll have to improve when he starts courting! But then again he could be right, as he was with Star.

Five years ago, Paul wanted a pup and after much coaxing and blackmail he got his way and we got Star. But a pup is a dog on the way, lovely for three or four weeks and then... the trouble! But five years later Paul still walks the dog before he sets off for school. Besides, Star has become a great favourite with all the family and if he needs to be taken for a walk, there is no shortage of volunteers.

I have experienced many great firsts: the first cry, the first, smile, the first gurgle, the first tooth, the first step, the first word, the first day at school, First Communion. I have experienced too the terrible twos. When cupboards, drawers, presses, boxes and fireplaces were explored or rummaged or vandalised, letters, cards, books were shredded and anything that moved or made a rattle was scattered. I had all these, three times over.

There were small things too that took me by surprise, like the day Paul, not yet three, went out the front door saying that he was going 'to play with my friend.' Yes I thought, they leave you!

Before that the back garden was enough.

They were busy, exciting, sometimes too exciting, eventful and satisfying times!

Down through the years I have had my share of good luck, I cannot say otherwise. Above all I have had the steadiness of Vincent. When I was eighteen I was out for fun, adventure, romance and excitement, and out there in front of me was a big exciting world which I was determined to greet with open arms. Vincent, with his manner cool and steadfast as a rock, did not appeal to me. Since then I have learned to appreciate his steadfast nature and to know my luck.

John, too, stood by me down all the years, never abandoned me when many others would have and for that he must always have my respect and admiration. Then there remains the Adult Literacy Programme in which I have spent half my life span already, my life sentence and my life line at the same time. As Wordsworth puts it:

> What though radiance, once so bright,
> Be now forever taken from my sight,
> We will, grieve not, but rather find
> Strength in what remains behind.

'Was I embarrassing you tonight?' I would sometimes ask Vincent after some gathering where husbands were expected to be accompanied by their wives.

'Yes,' he would answer in his usual undramatic way.

'Was I embarrassing to you when we first went out together?'

'Yes,' he would say again never lifting his eyes from his newspaper.

I know once more that the essence of myself is still the same! I know too that he too knows the same. No one can have everything but I know that I have what I most wanted in life: to be loved and to love others in return.

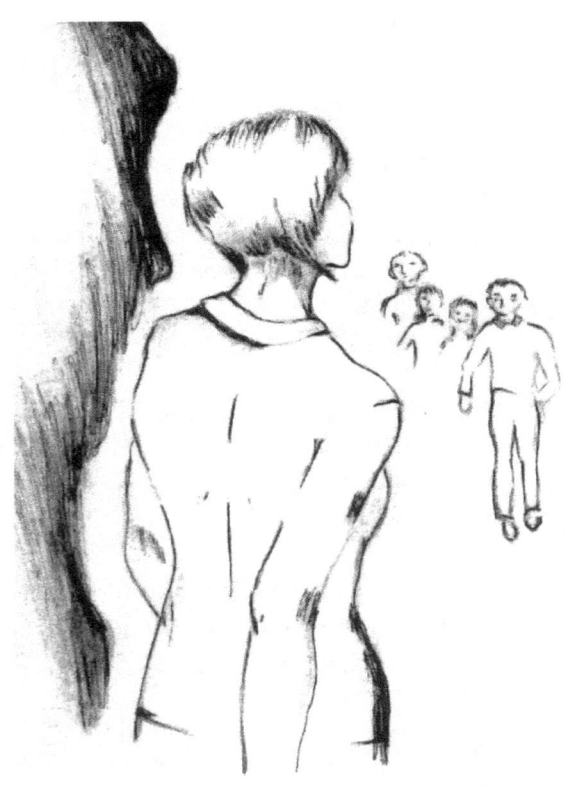

Postscript to 2015 edition

It is now 16 years since I wrote the print edition of my book. I am still enjoying life though I am more physically disabled. The ability to ride a bicycle is now a distant happy memory. I have less power on my right side which affects my walking. When I have needed to seek medical care I have found the staff to be more than willing to assist me. Finding the right words is an ongoing struggle. I continued to attend adult literacy classes for some years but these are no longer available to me.

Vincent and I were able to spend a year in South Africa doing voluntary work in 2006/07 which was one of the highlights of my life. Vincent had taken early retirement and we lived in a Camphill Community which has a residential and day school for children with learning difficulties. Our children were away from home and each was able to visit us over the year which made the separation bearable. I assisted in the Kindergarten and helped with the care of the children.

I still live in the small community of Killyclogher, near Omagh and have the support of kind family and friends. Our children are a delight to us. They have grown into thoughtful, caring adults seeking to make a contribution to the world.

Dympna Brogan

February 2015